RAW FOODS

FOR BUSY PEOPLE

Simple and Machine Free
Recipes for Every Day

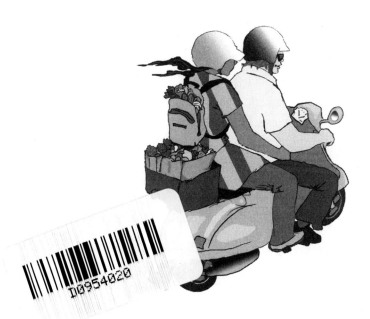

by Jordan Maerin

This book is dedicated to
The three people who got me started:

Raymond Francis, MSc, RNC
Nancy Gordon, LCSW
Aaron Howard

Cover Design: Vanesa Duran Christman
Illustrations: Bernadine Saint-Auguste

ISBN: 0-9774858-0-3
Second Edition, 2005
Printed in the USA

Acknowledgements:
Thanks to everyone who encouraged and inspired me and gave me
good ideas and feedback, including: Rob Titus, Aaron Howard,
Raymond Francis, Brian Anderson, Kimberly Dark, Nancy Gordon,
Chris O'Loughlin, the entire staff of Nature's First Law, and all those
who participated in the book's pre-sale. And most of all to my wife,
LaDawn, for her unwavering support and faith.

Disclaimer:
The responsibility for any adverse detoxification effects or
consequences resulting from the use of any suggestions described
hereafter lies not with the author or distributors of this book. This
book is not intended as medical advice. By following any suggested
dietary program, you are prescribing for yourself, which is your right.

TABLE OF CONTENTS

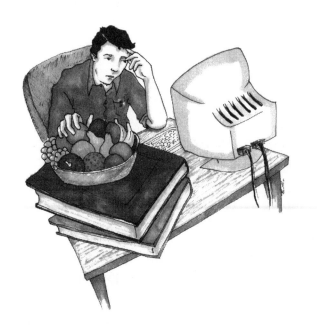

RAW FOODS FOR BUSY PEOPLE

PREFACE

Like a growing number of enthusiastically healthy people all over the world, switching to a raw food diet has given me a new lease on life!

At the age of 36 I was already experiencing signs of "aging", like widespread joint and back pain, chronic gum infections, constant indigestion and lack of energy. I felt like a wind-up toy that was winding inexorably *down*. I expected that I was just getting older and that my ailments would slowly worsen as I aged.

Culturally speaking, we often take this kind of physical deterioration for granted. How often have we shared "over the hill" jokes with our friends and family members?

Then I discovered the book *Never Be Sick Again* by Raymond Francis, M.Sc., R.N.C., and I suddenly had a glimpse into different possibilities. I came to see that the aches and pains I had been experiencing are not natural after all, though they are definitely, and tragically, the norm.

I subsequently discovered the writings of Dr. Norman Walker and Nature's First Law, and I was on my way to Paradise Health.

The high quantity of raw foods I've been eating is, in effect, new information for my body, which is speaking to me more loudly now that it knows I'm listening. In fact, I have come to prefer and *love* raw foods! Consequently, I've been learning about the processes of detoxification, and I am ever so grateful to people who make colon hygiene their priority and life's work. Thank you!

I have the energy of an adolescent again, and am enjoying a spiritual and emotional renaissance. I have expanded my expectations for my life, and for every single day I live. No more joint pains, gum infections, or indigestion. No more sinus headaches either, and sunburns are a thing of the past. Not only do I no longer feel sluggish, but exercising has become effortless, and I need much less sleep now than I used to. Cleansing my colon has relieved a lifetime of excruciating menstrual cramps for me, as well as the lower back aches I have suffered with for over a decade.

I had always been an enthusiastic vegetarian cook, both professionally and at home, so when I discovered raw foods I was excited to prepare and deliver them to my friends who were requesting them from me. I developed my raw repertoire by translating the recipes I had been using for years into raw versions, and then I studied gourmet raw recipe books and learned some new tricks. En route, I made great friends with my brand new machines: my food processor, dehydrator, juicer and Saladacco spiralizer.

After almost a year of preparing gourmet raw foods and working at my delivery business fulltime, however, I realized that I missed the simplicity of raw foods. Furthermore, I realized that most people wouldn't be able to spend the kind of time and energy I had been spending preparing raw gourmet foods every day of the week. Realizing that, I immediately made it my priority to develop a more simple and efficient daily routine for preparing tasty raw foods. My own return to a more simple raw diet has been very enjoyable for me, and it is my intention to help others create a simple raw food repertoire that they can maintain for the long run.

This book represents a compromise between simplicity and variety, ease and creativity. May it help you and your family on your path to Paradise Health!

INTRODUCTION

Let's face it. Busy people do not like to prepare food. We generally eat out. A lot.

If you want to eat raw foods but do not want to prepare anything yourself, then you'll subsist on fresh raw fruit and frequent your local salad bars. And if you're lucky, you'll live near a raw restaurant. End of story.

However, there are many easy ways to enjoy more variety while eating raw foods. In this book, I discuss strategies for eating out; direct you to some mail order resources for raw prepared foods; and, yes, encourage you to learn some very simple dishes that you can prepare for yourself.

Even the busiest people enjoy some variety in the foods they eat, especially over the long run. Helping you achieve Paradise Health, happily and conveniently, is what this book is all about.

I had two reasons for writing this book.

First, I want to remove the last vestige of an excuse for you to resist embracing the raw food diet: the prep time factor.

Secondly, I want to inspire you to become as comfortably functional preparing raw foods in your kitchen as you ever have been preparing cooked foods (maybe even more so!).

Let me give you an example of what I mean. Imagine wanting to prepare a grilled cheese sandwich. Do you refer to a cookbook to find out how much butter you should use on the bread? Do you get out your scale and ask your guest exactly how many ounces of cheese they want on their sandwich? Do you rely on a thermometer to tell you when your skillet is ready to receive the sandwich? Do you again consult a cookbook to find out exactly how long the sandwich should remain on the hot skillet before flipping it to the other side? Of course not!

Instead, you easily assemble the ingredients, eyeball the amount of butter and cheese, throw the sandwich onto the skillet when you're ready, and then peek underneath the bottom piece of bread to determine when you want to flip it.

These have become easy, comfortable rituals, whatever we've learned to do in our kitchens over the course of our lifetimes. It's an ease that we take for granted, until the day we discover a whole new way of eating, like the raw food diet. A new direction like this seems like a curve ball, a speed bump. Suddenly, we feel that the rules have changed, the restrictions multiplied, the machinery become unfamiliar.

With the help of this book, you'll discover that raw food preparation takes much less time than you'd thought. And I've put in some of the time and energy for you, by translating, compiling and creating some very simple recipes, and consolidating them into types that will be easy for you to remember and duplicate.

With this book as your guide, you'll never again come home after an exhausting day and think, "I don't have the time and energy to make something healthy to eat."

Think of this book as your launching pad, as you discover the ease and comfort of preparing the most nutritious foods that nature has to offer, within the comfort of your own home.

Easy, natural, simple. This is the road to Paradise Health.

CHAPTER 1:
THE ABC'S OF RAW

If you've picked up this book out of curiosity, you've probably already heard something about the healing and energizing powers of raw foods.

Raymond Francis, M.Sc., R.N.C., in his book, *Never Be Sick Again: Health is a Choice Learn How to Choose It*, explains why raw foods heal. Human disease manifests in many forms, but it has only one underlying cause: cellular malfunction. Cellular malfunction, in turn, has only two causes: deficiency and toxicity. Since cooking your food destroys vital nutrients and enzymes, the only way to give your cells all the nutrients they need and protect them from substances that are toxic or unusable, is to eat a diet that is at least 80% raw, and 100% whole and organic.

The evidence Raymond Francis presents includes his own recovery from near-fatal liver failure and chemical hepatitis, as well as an inspiring look at the healthiest peoples on the planet, including the disease-free Hunza people of the Himalayas.

Many Natural Hygienists and colon therapists agree with Raymond. The naturally high fiber content of raw foods is the key to a healthy digestive system and colon, and therefore to the absorption of optimum nutrition for every cell in your body. For more information, read *The Natural Hygiene Handbook* by the American Natural Hygiene Society, and *Colon Health: Key to a Vibrant Life* by Dr. Norman Walker.

ENZYMES = ENERGY

Living foods come stocked with their own digestive enzymes. When we eat lifeless, enzyme-less foods, our bodies must create digestive enzymes, pulling energy from other areas and organs of the body, which is why eating cooked foods creates a feeling of lethargy, or the feeling that you want to take a nap. Eating raw will help keep your energy naturally elevated.

Conserving the body's enzyme resources is particularly important if you need those resources to heal from a serious illness.

BLOOD TYPES AND ALKALINITY

Natural carnivores have acidic blood and short colons. Human beings have alkaline blood and long colons, like other plant-eaters. Eating cooked and processed foods and animal products raises our acidity unnaturally, which in turn causes degeneration and disease. This is true for all humans, regardless of blood type.

To alkalinize your blood, rely on raw plant foods, especially fresh citrus fruits, leafy greens and almonds. For more information, read *Become Younger* by Dr. Norman Walker or *Rainbow Green Live Food Cuisine* by Gabriel Cousens, M.D.

BEYOND PROTEIN

The idea that protein comes only from meat and dairy products is a myth. Proteins are basically amino acids, which are present in all raw foods, especially wheatgrass juice, alfalfa sprouts, and sprouted sunflower seeds.

Raw bodybuilders, like Stephen Arlin, author of *Raw Power!: Building Strength and Muscle Naturally,* list these quality sources of protein: heavy greens, like romaine lettuce and kale, as well as avocadoes, olives, coconuts, and flax seeds.

SLOW OR FAST?

The pace at which you'll transition to raw foods will depend on whether you're currently in a health crisis, in which case you'll probably want to transition quickly.

A slow transition is generally more comfortable, and it's a miraculous process listening to our bodies as they change.

For more information, I recommend the book *Conscious Eating* by Gabriel Cousens, M.D. The lack of immediate motivation for those of us who are not in emergency situations, however, can be frustrating. It's tempting to put off our commitment to raw foods to a hundred or a thousand tomorrows.

If you want to make a quick transition to raw foods because of immediate health concerns, hold onto your motivation with both hands; read *12 Steps to Raw Foods: How to End Your Addiction to Cooked Food* by Victoria Boutenko; and consider enjoying a retreat at a raw foods healing center, several of which are listed in the back of this book.

Another good book for people facing motivational issues in emergency situations is *Man's Search for Meaning* by Victor Frankl.

HOW RAW IS RAW?

There are many different philosophies of health and spirituality that can pique a person's interest in a raw plant food diet. Each of the health systems listed below encourages a diet consisting of at least 75% raw, living plant foods. Their differences lie in whether they recommend eating any cooked food at all, and if so, what kinds and why.

100% Raw Plant Food Diet - The path to discovering how truly healthy you can be. Devotees enjoy a completely mucusless and alkaline physical state. Books: *The Sunfood Diet Success System* by David Wolfe and *12 Steps to Raw Foods* by Victoria Boutenko.

Hippocrates Diet - A 100% raw plant food diet, focusing on maximum enzyme sources like sprouts, wheatgrass juice and fermented foods like fresh sauerkraut. Books: *The Hippocrates Diet and Health Program* by Dr. Ann Wigmore and *The Living Foods Lifestyle* by Brenda Cobb.

Natural Hygiene - Primarily a raw plant food diet, with cooked complex starches, like potatoes, yams, lentils and legumes, to increase calorie intake. Books: *The Natural Hygiene Handbook* by the American Natural Hygiene Society, and any book by Dr. Herbert M. Shelton.

Essene Diet - Based on *The Essene Gospel of Peace*, God gave us to eat raw seeds, fruit, herbs and milk. That is, milk which is unpasteurized and from healthy animals.

Macrobiotic-Raw Diet - Focus on raw plant foods, with miso, seaweed, and possibly brown rice and soy products included. The focus is on enzymes, and B-complex vitamins. Book: *Dining in the Raw* by Rita Romano.

Hunza Diet - An 80% raw plant food diet, with some cooked whole grains, and healthy meat and eggs included. A practical approach based on the long-lived, disease-free people of the Hunza culture. Book: *Never Be Sick Again* by Raymond Francis, M.Sc., R.N.C.

Temporary Raw Diet - Raw foods and juices are very effective for purposes of detoxification and colon cleansing. Books: *Juice Fasting and Detoxification* by Steve Meyerowitz and *Cleanse and Purify Thyself* by Richard Anderson.

THE SKINNY ON DETOXIFICATION

When we regularly ingest processed foods, meat and dairy products, our lymphatic systems become overloaded, or congested, leaving excess toxins to remain rampant in the blood and in the digestive system where they cause chronic illnesses and diseased colons.

Raw foods help our digestive systems to heal, which allows our lymphatic systems to discharge these congestive toxins. This process can be uncomfortable.

Symptoms of detoxification include a temporary loss of energy, headaches, nausea or diarrhea. Some people will re-experience childhood illnesses. If you experience low energy or bowel irregularities over a long period of time, you may have an overgrowth of yeast, or Candida, in your intestines.

If eating raw foods makes you feel ill, find a supportive health practitioner who can help you to detox more slowly, and read *The Detox Miracle Sourcebook* by Robert Morse, N.D.

HABITS AND ALLERGIES

As you embark on your own brand of raw diet, be as open as you can be to challenging your previous, habitual tastes. Sweet and salty flavors dominate in the standard American diet, but as Deepak Chopra reminds us, there are six flavors of health: sweet, salty, bitter, pungent, astringent and sour.

Before I'd started eating primarily raw foods, I had disliked avocadoes and olives immensely. Since these are two important raw sources of essential fatty acids, I challenged myself to give each of them another honest try. Lo and behold, I took to raw olives immediately, and I can now say that I miss avocadoes if I go a couple of days without them. I now even enjoy spicy foods, where I was previously very sensitive to them and disliked peppers in general. Let miracles happen.

Be open to the possibility that your food allergies will change as well. Many people find that as they eat more raw foods and detoxify their bodies, their food allergies, as well as environmental and pet allergies, will disappear. If your allergies are potentially severe or life threatening, however, you may want to work with a health practitioner to determine when you can experiment again with the foods to which you've been allergic.

CONVENIENCE FOODS

Raw-food-to-go is a great timesaving option.

Besides fresh fruit, which is the ultimate convenience food, you can also buy flax seed crackers, raw energy bars and dried fruit at most health food stores now. In some states, you can buy unpasteurized juices in the bottle; for instance, bottled orange and grapefruit juices can legally be sold in California without being pasteurized.

If the stores near you don't carry what you want, you can request them. Fresh salad bars are also convenient and quick, so keep these in mind, including those located in mainstream grocery stores in your area.

If needed, there are companies who can ship convenient raw food items to you. Several are listed in the back of this book.

EATING OUT

Raw restaurants are popping up in cities all over the country and the world, and an increasing number of vegetarian restaurants, and health food stores and delis, are becoming raw food conscious. You can help your local restaurants and delis through the learning curve by turning them on to a few simple raw recipe books.

In lieu of raw friendly businesses, many mainstream restaurants offer fresh-squeezed orange juice, fruit plates, creative large dinner salads or salad bars, as well as innovative salad dressings. For a healthier salad dressing, you can bring a small bottle of flax oil with you to restaurants and request fresh lemon wedges. I usually request fresh avocado slices for my salads, which adds some creaminess. In the summertime, some restaurants offer cold, fresh soups, like gazpacho.

Find out where the fresh juice bars are in your area, and include them on your daily route.

Another tactic I use includes bringing my own flax crackers to Mexican restaurants so I can enjoy fresh guacamole and salsa. At Japanese restaurants, I may order miso soup with my green salad. At Jewish delis, I eat fresh pickles and marinated coleslaws and salads.

Once you start looking at the world through "raw eyes," you'll get more creative and feel more comfortable making special requests when you eat out.

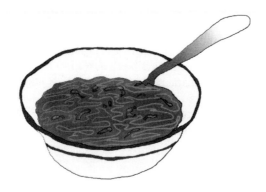

CHAPTER 2:
USING THIS BOOK

Over half of the recipes in this book include machine-free options. Some of you may wonder why.

First, machines can be intimidating for raw food beginners. The idea of purchasing and using unfamiliar machinery can be an additional barrier to the already overwhelming project of switching to raw foods.

Secondly, it is unnecessarily time-consuming to assemble, use and clean up after machines.

Thirdly, noisy machinery is contraindicated when one is pursuing a simpler diet and lifestyle.

Therefore, I have structured each chapter as a progression, starting with the simplest recipes, and ending with a recipe that includes a more advanced concept in raw food preparation, like sprouting or using a nut-milk bag.

Each recipe that can be made without a machine will include this symbol:

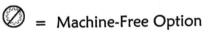 = Machine-Free Option

Likewise, if a machine is necessary or optional for a recipe, you will see one or more of these symbols:

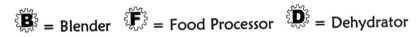 = Blender   = Food Processor   = Dehydrator

For machine-free food preparation, I suggest you have on hand a whisk, a mandoline or manual grater, a manual citrus juicer, and a mortar and pestle if you love pesto. If you're interested in quiet, electricity-free machines, you can purchase a hand crank blender and a manual wheatgrass juicer.

The number one machine I recommend for busy people is a Vita-Mix, since being able to make large batches of smoothies and soups is a real time-saver. The number two machine I recommend is a dehydrator because you can make large batches of convenience foods, suited to your own tastes.

INGREDIENTS

If some of the ingredients in this book are unfamiliar to you, you can scan the list below for descriptions, including simple tips on how to choose the highest quality ingredients.

Agave nectar: A sweet syrup from a common desert plant.

Bragg's liquid aminos: A healthy salt alternative that is not fermented like soy sauces are.

Carob Powder: A powdered cacao substitute. Choose raw.

Cashews: Buy hand-shelled, truly raw cashews, if possible.

Date sugar: Granulated sugar made from dried dates.

Flax seeds: Small brown or golden seeds, which are high in healthy essential oils. They make great crunchy crackers when dehydrated. Flax oil is great on salads.

Honey: Buy raw, unfiltered honey, and make sure it hasn't been diluted with corn syrup, like many commercial brands are, even though it doesn't say so on the label.

Maca: A powdered nutritious root from Peru that gives a malted flavor to smoothies and beverages.

Maple syrup: Buy the 100% pure variety. Though not uncooked, it is often the easiest plant-based sweetener to find.

Miso: Miso is a salty, fermented soybean product. Though it's cooked, it's also packed with healthy enzymes.

Nama Shoyu: Unpasteurized soy sauce by Ohsawa.

Oils: Always use cold-pressed, unrefined, organic oils.

Olive Oil: Studies show that 96% of the "100% Extra Virgin Olive Oil" sold in the U.S. is *NOT!* For more information, call or visit the website for Beyond Health.

Olives: Raw olives are those that have been dried or cured without pasteurized, acidic vinegars.

Salt: Sea salt is rich in minerals. Try Celtic or Himalayan.

Spices: Organic are better. Sun-dried are best.

Tahini: Sesame butter used in popular Middle Eastern dishes like hummus and falafel. Choose raw.

Vinegar: Raw apple cider vinegar is the healthiest unpasteurized, alkalizing vinegar.

Young coconut: Also called a Thai coconut, this is the one covered with tough white fibers. Carefully chop open with a large knife or machete to reach the tender meat and water.

Throughout this book, I often suggest timesaving shortcuts, such as using garlic and ginger powders. However, there is really no substitute for fresh garlic and ginger, when you have the time and energy to prepare it.

If you're avoiding fermented foods, you'll want to substitute fresh lemon juice for vinegar, and Bragg's liquid aminos for Nama Shoyu in these recipes, and you'll want to skip the miso entirely.

WARMING YOUR FOOD

The temperature at which a significant amount of vital enzymes are destroyed in natural foods is somewhere between 108 and 119 degrees.

When warming liquids like soups and sauces, use a double boiler so that the temperature will rise slowly. Stir often, and either use a thermometer or heat just until the liquid is warm to the touch.

When warming entrees, a dehydrator is the safest way to reheat food. About an hour at 105 degrees, or a little higher, will do. Another option is to use a slightly warmed oven.

Microwaves destroy enzymes, so use sparingly, or never.

For further guidance, see *Warming Up to Living Foods* by Elisa Markowitz.

A DAILY MENU

For those of you who aren't sure what a daily raw menu would look like, here's a sample, with plenty of options:

BREAKFAST:
Fresh grapefruit or other fresh fruit, OR
A fruit smoothie or pudding, OR
Hot tea with a Sweet Seed Bar or Nut Butter Cookie

LUNCH:
Small green salad, or coleslaw, WITH
Marinated Vegetables or Waldorf Salad, OR
Pâté or Guacamole with Flax Crackers, OR
Soup or Rellenos or other raw entrée

MID-AFTERNOON:
Fresh vegetable juice, or Jordan's Power Shake

DINNER:
A large green salad, packed with garnishes, olives, avocadoes, sprouts, cucumbers, tomatoes, etc.

EVENING:
A shake, smoothie or fresh fruit, OR
A dessert, energy bar, or cookie

Since our digestive systems are strongest at mid-day, I enjoy my more elaborate recipes then. If your schedule doesn't allow for it, or if you enjoy more creative meals in the evenings, you'll probably want to swap my Afternoon suggestions with my Evening suggestions.

A BUSY WEEK

Here's an example of how a busy person can organize a workweek to support a raw diet:

SUNDAY:
Make prepared-ahead foods, like a salad dressing and garnish, a pate, a ready-to-use marinade, Ice Dream, a fruit dip, etc.

MONDAY – WEDNESDAY:
Rely on prepared-ahead food items.

THURSDAY – FRIDAY:
Rely on grab-and-go food items, like fresh fruit, oil and vinegar for your salads, Guacamole, smoothies and quick soups.

SATURDAY:
Take some time to prepare and enjoy gourmet recipes, like Rellenos, Cottage Pie, Nori Rolls, Refried Almonds, etc.

ONE SUNDAY PER MONTH:
Stack your dehydrator with foods you can enjoy all month.

RECIPES

RAW FOODS FOR BUSY PEOPLE

CHAPTER 3:
EXCITING SALADS

Green salads and fresh fruit form a strong dietary base for us humans. However, for the vast majority of us, our palates have received constant stimulation from such a wide variety of cooked foods that the switch to eating a large green salad or two every day can take some getting used to. It can seem boring, or repetitive, at first. That is, until the sigh of relief your body gives you every time you eat raw fruits and greens overpowers that desire for the cooked, processed foods of yore.

Well, it's time for greener pastures! This chapter lists some exciting ways to turn your green salads into fields of adventure. If you make a week's worth of a different raw salad dressing and salad garnish each weekend, you'll find yourself looking forward to your salads every day of the week.

Making your own salad dressings will help you to avoid refined sugars, acidic vinegars and processed oils. Of course, simple flaxseed or olive oil, with raw apple cider vinegar or fresh lemon juice, makes the most effortless salad dressing.

Recipes for coleslaws and Waldorf salad are also included in this chapter, as is a brief introduction to sprouting techniques.

For fruit salad dressings, please see page 57 in the "Dip This, Dip That" chapter.

RAW FOODS FOR BUSY PEOPLE

⊘ ⚙ Ⓑ SIMPLE VINAIGRETTES

Keep this one handy. It makes a great marinade too.

BASIC VINAIGRETTE:

1 cup extra virgin olive oil

½ cup raw cider or balsamic vinegar, or a mixture

3 cloves garlic, minced, or ½ tsp. garlic powder

2 Tb. honey or agave syrup

1 tsp. each salt and black pepper

2 tsp. each dried oregano and basil

Dried chili peppers (optional)

CREAMY VINAIGRETTE:

Add 3-4 stalks of celery to the Basic Vinaigrette recipe

RASPBERRY VINAIGRETTE:

½ Basic Vinaigrette recipe

1 pint raspberries, fresh or frozen

½ cup orange juice

1 chopped scallion

MARINATED MUSHROOMS OR CHERRY TOMATOES:

Mushrooms or tomatoes, plus Basic Vinaigrette to coat

A Basic Vinaigrette can be assembled in any kind of a jar, and then shaken before each use. For the Raspberry or Creamy Vinaigrette, you'll need to use a blender.

Marinate cherry tomatoes or mushrooms, or any other vegetable of your choice, in the Basic Vinaigrette for three hours at room temperature, stirring often, or overnight in the refrigerator, stirring occasionally. Enjoy as a salad garnish, or as munchies at any time of day.

⊘ ⚙ TAHINI DRESSING

Tahini makes a deliciously rich dressing for salads.

2/3 cup tahini

1 cup water

¼ cup lemon or orange juice

1 clove garlic, minced, or ¼ tsp. garlic powder

¼ cup chopped parsley

1 tsp. salt and a pinch of cayenne

1 pitted date (optional)

BELL PEPPER SALAD:

2 cups diced bell peppers, mixed colors

1 cup chopped cauliflower

½ cup chopped red onion

1 stalk celery, chopped

1/3 cup Tahini Dressing

2 Tb. Italian Seasoning

If using a whisk to mix the dressing, make sure the tahini is at room temperature. For a super smooth dressing, use a blender.

For the Bell Pepper Salad, simply toss and serve.

⊘ ⚙ INSTANT RANCH DRESSING

You can whip this up in two minutes flat.

1 cup cashew butter

½ cup water

3 Tb. lemon juice

1 tsp. raw cider vinegar

Pinch of salt

1 tsp. Italian seasoning or dried dill

1 clove garlic

1 stalk celery

Combine all ingredients in a blender and whip until smooth and creamy.

For a machine-free version, replace the salt and celery stalk with a bit of celery salt, and make sure your cashew butter is at room temperature.

⊘ 🄱 AVOCADO DRESSING

Creates a salad packed with essential oils.

2 ripe avocadoes

3-4 Tb. lemon juice

1 clove garlic

1 medium cucumber, peeled

¼ cup chopped scallions OR red onion

1 Tb. Italian seasoning OR dried dill

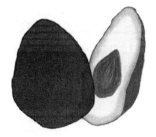

AVOCADO TOMATO DRESSING:

Add 1 ripe tomato

Blend all ingredients together, adding water to desired consistency.

Avocadoes can easily be whipped to a creamy and smooth consistency without a blender, so if you use a whisk, simply replace the cucumber with enough water to thin.

JORDAN'S SLACKER SALAD

This is my dinner when I feel really lazy.

1 chopped tomato

1 handful of raw olives

1 chopped avocado (optional)

Basic Vinaigrette Dressing (page 21)

Toss and enjoy.

COOL MINT SALAD

Cool, light and refreshing, all year round.

1 cup chopped cucumbers

1 cup chopped tomatoes

1/3 cup chopped fresh mint

¼ cup chopped parsley

2 Tb. lemon juice

1 Tb. olive oil

¼ cup sprouted sunflower seeds (page 32) (optional)

RAWESOME TABOULI:

Increase chopped parsley to 1 cup

Add ½ recipe Sprouted Lentil Salad (page 32) minus vinegar

Toss all ingredients and allow to marinate in the refrigerator at least one hour, stirring often.

⊘ CHINESE CELERY SALAD

A taste of the Orient.

6 stalks celery

1 cup mushrooms of your choice (optional)

2 Tb. Nama Shoyu

1 Tb. raw cider vinegar

1 Tb. sesame oil

1 tsp. fresh grated ginger, or ¼ tsp. ginger powder

Pinch of salt

Sliced Chinese cabbage, and shredded carrots

Thinly slice the celery, and toss with mushrooms, tamari, vinegar, lemon juice, ginger and salt. Allow to marinate for 3 hours at room temperature, stirring often, or overnight in the refrigerator, stirring occasionally.

Serve on a bed of Chinese cabbage, and garnish with shredded carrots.

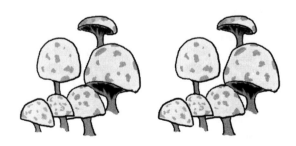

⊘ CAULIFLOWER ORANGE SALAD

The best recipe I ever translated from Betty Crocker.

½ small head of cauliflower, chopped

½ bell pepper, chopped

½ cup chopped green beans or broccoli

1 ½ cups mandarin orange segments

3 Tb. lemon juice

3 Tb. flaxseed or olive oil

1 tsp. maple syrup or honey

½ tsp. orange zest

Salt and black pepper to taste

Serve on a bed of spinach, and garnish with chives

Toss all ingredients and allow to marinate for three hours at room temperature, stirring often, or overnight in the refrigerator, stirring occasionally.

For a more portable version, skip the green beans or broccoli, and add 1-2 cups of chopped spinach, allowing it to marinate and reduce within the salad.

⊘ ⚙F LIGHT SUMMER COLE SLAW

Click your heels three times, and you'll have it memorized.

3 cups shredded green and/or red cabbage

1 cup shredded carrots

2 celery stalks, thinly sliced

2 Tb. chopped parsley

½ cup pecans or walnuts, or nuts of your choice

¼ cup sesame oil

2 Tb. cider vinegar

½ tsp. garlic powder

½ cup sun-dried tomatoes, soaked 15 minutes, chopped (opt.)

1 tsp. fennel or poppy seeds (optional)

Salt and black pepper to taste

Slice the cabbage and carrots by hand, or use a mandoline. If you want to finely shred the cabbage and carrots, use the shredding blade on a food processor.

Toss all ingredients and allow to marinate at least one hour, stirring often.

SWEET RED CABBAGE

Kids of all ages will love this.

4 cups red cabbage, thinly sliced

2 pears or apples, sliced

3 green onions, sliced

1 carrot, grated

½ cup raisins or currants

4 Tb. apple juice, or 2Tb. agave syrup

3 Tb. olive oil

1 Tb. raw cider vinegar

½ tsp. dry mustard (optional)

Salt and pepper to taste

Toss all ingredients together and marinate for 2 hours at room temperature, stirring often, or overnight in the refrigerator, stirring occasionally.

Ⓞ Ⓑ Ⓕ CREAMY PINEAPPLE SALADS

A sweet, tropical treat.

CREAMY PINEAPPLE SAUCE:

¼ cup cashew or macadamia butter

¼ cup pineapple juice

1 Tb. lemon juice

½ Tb. olive oil

2 tsp. dried dill

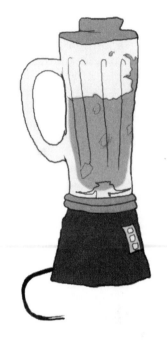

CREAMY PINEAPPLE COLESLAW:

2 cups shredded green cabbage

½ cup shredded carrots

1 cup pineapple chunks

2 Tb. chopped parsley

Creamy Pineapple Sauce

Salt and pepper to taste

PINEAPPLE WALDORF SALAD:

1 chopped apple

½ cup pineapple chunks

3 stalks celery, sliced

3-4 scallions, chopped

½ cup walnuts or pecans

¼ cup parsley, chopped

Creamy Pineapple Sauce

Salt to taste

Whisk or blend sauce ingredients together. If using a whisk, make sure the nut butter is at room temperature. If using a blender, add the dill last and gently pulse blend. For very fine coleslaw, you can shred the cabbage with a food processor.

Toss all ingredients, and serve fresh. Waldorf Salad is great served on a bed of greens.

⊘ F FESTIVE SALAD GARNISHES

These are great topped with avocado slices.

4 cups shredded carrots, beets and/or Daikon radish

¼ cup each minced scallions and parsley

One of the marinades from Chapter 4, OR

Sour Cream (page 39), OR

TANGY MARINADE:

¼ cup orange juice

2 Tb. lemon juice

1 Tb. olive oil

1 Tb. orange zest

Pinch of cayenne

It's easiest to make a week's worth of these salad garnishes by using the shredding blade on a food processor, but a mandoline or hand shredder will work just as well.

Toss all ingredients and allow to marinate at least one hour, stirring often.

Serve as a garnish with a green salad.

⊘ SPROUTS DEMYSTIFIED

The trick is in the timing.

1 cup seeds or legumes soaked in 4 cups water

SUNFLOWER SEEDS: Soak 8-12 hours, air dry for 2-4 hours
GARBANZOS/LENTILS: Soak 8-12 hours, air dry 2-3 days

Sprouting is easy, in concept. The challenge for busy people is to remember that something's sprouting, and to drain or rinse the seeds or legumes in a timely manner.

Soak your seeds or legumes in the refrigerator overnight, then rinse well. Leave them in the strainer or colander to allow them to air dry, re-rinsing the legumes once per day. Legumes will be ready to use when they sprout a tail about ¼ inch long.

Sprouted seeds and legumes are great on green salads. Use sunflower seeds for making Versatile Pates (page 59), or use lentils in the Sprouted Lentil Salad (below).

⊘ SPROUTED LENTIL SALAD

Use plenty of tomato, and serve with a green salad.

1 ½ cups sprouted lentils

1 ½ cups chopped tomatoes

½ cup each chopped onion and bell pepper

2 Tb. lemon juice or raw cider vinegar

4 Tb. olive oil

1 tsp. honey or maple syrup

Salt to taste

Toss sprouted lentils with the rest of the ingredients, and allow to marinate at least one hour.

Serve as a garnish with a green salad, or use in the Rawsome Tabouli recipe on page 26.

CHAPTER 4:
MARINADES
AND OTHER
WET STUFF

These recipes are my favorites because they punctuate the ease and simplicity of raw foods. Chop up a batch of your favorite veggies, add a marinade, and munch on them for days.

Here's the easiest way to marinate: Simply seal your vegetables and marinade of choice in an air-tight container; leave it on your counter for a few hours; and shake it up whenever you walk by. Or, if you leave the container in your refrigerator, you can give it a shake when you go in there for something else.

Another bonus: when you use marinades that include acidic ingredients, like lemon juice, Nama Shoyu, or cider vinegar, the vegetables will soften as they "simmer" in the marinade. This is true especially of mushrooms, broccoli, and greens like spinach or bok choy.

Most of these recipes can be made without machinery, so the clean up is almost nil. Remember your whisk? Dust it off, honey!

RAW FOODS FOR BUSY PEOPLE

⊘ SIMPLEST MARINADE

Memorize it. Use it. Play with it!

3 Tb. Nama Shoyu

1-2 cloves garlic

1 Tb. fresh lime or lemon juice

1 tsp. honey or agave syrup

Black pepper or cayenne

1 Tb. unrefined sesame or olive oil

POLYNESIAN MARINADE:

Use fresh pineapple juice and chunks in place of citrus

MEDITERRANEAN MARINADE:

Omit Nama Shoyu

Increase olive oil to ¼ cup and lemon juice to 3 Tb.

Add 1 tsp. oregano, and chopped olives to taste

Whisk ingredients together. Marinate vegetables of your choice for 2-3 hours at room temperature, stirring often, or overnight in the refrigerator, stirring occasionally.

Serve atop fresh, crunchy bean sprouts, or make Vegetable Kabobs (page 66).

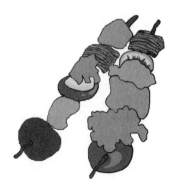

⊘ ⚙️ ALMOND BUTTER MARINADE

You can make this rich sauce as spicy as you like.

½ cup each raw almond butter and water

¼ cup Nama Shoyu

¼ cup honey, or chopped dates

3-4 cloves garlic

1 tsp. raw apple cider vinegar

Crushed red pepper, cayenne, and sea salt to taste

Whisk or blend all ingredients together. Toss with vegetables of your choice and marinate for 2-3 hours at room temperature, stirring often, or overnight in the refrigerator, stirring occasionally.

If using dates, you'll want to use a blender.

Serve as is, or atop fresh, crunchy bean sprouts.

⊘ MOROCCAN MARINADE

A blend of exotic flavors.

¼ cup olive or sesame oil

3 tsp. coriander

1 ½ tsp. cinnamon

2 Tb. fresh lemon juice

2 tsp. honey or agave syrup (optional)

1 tsp. dried orange peel or saffron (optional)

Whisk the marinade and toss with vegetables of your choice. Allow vegetables to marinate for 2-3 hours at room temperature, stirring often, or overnight in the refrigerator, stirring occasionally.

I suggest including fresh chopped tomatoes and bell peppers when using this sauce. It's also a good marinade for shredded yam.

⊘ CURRIED APPLE MARINADE

This sauce is great with carrots, cauliflower and bell peppers.

½ cup apple juice, preferably fresh

2 Tb. unrefined sesame or olive oil

2-4 Tb. diced onion

1 tsp. garam masala or curry powder

¼ tsp. each dry mustard and black pepper

Cayenne to taste, or minced hot peppers

Combine all ingredients. Toss with vegetables and allow to marinate for 2-3 hours, stirring often, or overnight in the refrigerator, stirring occasionally.
    Serve atop fresh, crunchy bean sprouts, or make Vegetable Kabobs (page 66).

⊘ SZECHWAN MARINADE

This is a powerful sauce best made with rice wine.

¼ cup unrefined sesame oil

2-3 Tb. rice wine

2-3 Tb. Nama Shoyu

3 cloves garlic, or ½ tsp. garlic powder

1 tsp. dry mustard

½ tsp. crushed red pepper, or minced hot peppers

Whisk the ingredients together and toss with vegetables of your choice. Allow to marinate for 2-3 hours at room temperature, stirring often, or overnight in the refrigerator, stirring occasionally.
    Serve atop fresh, crunchy bean sprouts, or make Vegetable Kabobs (page 66).

⚙ MARINARA MARINADE

Try chopped zucchini, bell peppers and mushrooms with this sauce.

2 large tomatoes

2 Tb. olive oil

1 tsp. cider vinegar or lemon juice

2 Tb. Italian seasoning

1 small clove garlic

2-4 black olives, chopped (optional)

½ Tb. sweetener of choice (optional)

Salt to taste

PIZZA SAUCE: Add ½ cup sun-dried tomatoes, soaked 15 min.

SPAGHETTI: Serve Marinara Marinade over zucchini noodles

Blend all ingredients and toss with vegetables of your choice. Allow to marinate for 2-3 hours at room temperature, stirring often, or overnight in the refrigerator, stirring occasionally.

To make zucchini noodles, use a Saladacco or Spirooli spiralizer. The noodles can be warmed in a dehydrator for 30 minutes, or in a double boiler with the sauce.

Add sun-dried tomatoes for a smoother, richer sauce. Use as a pizza spread, with Italian Flax Crackers you can purchase or dehydrate yourself (page 68).

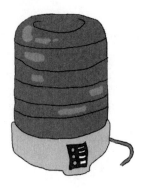

⊘ 🅱 CITRUS GINGER MARINADE

Fresh ginger makes this sauce exquisite.

½ cup orange or pineapple juice

¼ cup Nama Shoyu

1 Tb. fresh grated ginger

2-3 cloves garlic, or ½ tsp. garlic powder

1-2 Tb. honey or agave syrup

1 Tb. unrefined sesame oil

Whisk or blend the ingredients together and toss with vegetables of your choice. Allow to marinate for 2-3 hours at room temperature, stirring often, or overnight in the refrigerator, stirring occasionally.

Serve atop fresh, crunchy bean sprouts; dehydrate for Vegetable Kabobs (page 66); or use to make Asian Pate (page 59).

🅱 SOUR CREAM

A creamy classic with a smooth consistency.

1 cup raw cashews, soaked 30 minutes and drained

¼ cup lemon juice

½ stalk celery, peeled and chopped

Pinch of salt

1 scallion, chopped, to garnish (optional)

Blend cashews with lemon juice and a little water, if needed, until the nuts dissolve and a truly smooth consistency is reached. Scrape the sides of the blender with a spatula to aid in blending. Add the remaining ingredients.

Use to accompany Anything-You-Want Borscht (page 49), or Rawsome Rellenos (page 70).

⚙ PINEAPPLE BARBECUE SAUCE

Fresh and tangy. Accept no substitute.

1 cup chopped fresh tomatoes

½ cup sun-dried tomatoes, soaked 15 minutes, chopped

2 Tb. pineapple juice, plus ¼ cup pineapple chunks

¼ cup chopped onion

1 small clove garlic, or 1/8 tsp. garlic powder

¼ tsp. cayenne, or minced hot peppers

2 Tb. maple syrup, or to taste

2 Tb. olive or sesame oil

1 tsp. salt, or to taste

¼ tsp. each paprika and black pepper

Combine all ingredients, and blend until smooth.

Use to top off a batch of Vegetable Kabobs (page 66), or the Barbecue Portobello (below). It's also used as the base for Chunky Tomato Chili (page 48).

⊘ ⚙ BARBECUE PORTOBELLO

A hearty meal you can create to suit your tastes.

Vegetable Kabobs, made with chunks of Portobello (page 66)

Pineapple Barbecue Sauce (above)

Crispy Onion Toppers (page 66)

For a satisfying entrée, drizzle the Kabobs with Pineapple Barbecue Sauce, and garnish with Crispy Onion Toppers.

For a machine-free version, simply toss marinated vegetables and Portobello with fresh chopped tomato and pineapple chunks, and drizzle with a little maple syrup.

⊘ Ⓑ QUICKEST GRAVY

So simple, you'll wonder where it's been all your life.

¾ cup water

1 Tb. unpasteurized miso of your choice

2 Tb. raw almond butter or sesame tahini

1/8 tsp. garlic powder

Pinch of black pepper

Whisk or blend all ingredients together.
   If using a whisk, make sure the almond butter or tahini is at room temperature.
   Use over Vegetable Kabobs or instead of the Barbecue Sauce on the Barbecue Portobello (previous page). Or, pour it over a batch of the "Mashed Potatoes" that form the topping of the Cottage Pie (see below).

Ⓕ COTTAGE PIE

Marinated vegetables topped with "Mashed Potatoes".
The Queen Mother never had it so good!

2 cups total chopped broccoli, cauliflower and carrots

½ cup minced celery

¼ cup minced red onion

¼ cup chopped parsley

½ cup chopped spinach (optional)

2 Tb. each olive oil and Nama Shoyu

½ Tb. organic red wine

1 clove garlic, minced, or ¼ tsp. garlic powder

Pinch of black pepper or cayenne

¼ cup sun-dried tomatoes, soaked 15 minutes, chopped

"MASHED POTATOES":

2 cups chopped cauliflower

2/3 cup raw cashews or macadamias, soaked 30 min.

¼ cup lemon juice

2 Tb. olive oil

1 clove garlic, or ¼ tsp. garlic powder

1 tsp. rosemary or Italian seasoning

Salt and pepper to taste

Marinate vegetables in olive oil, Nama Shoyu, red wine, garlic and black pepper for at least 1 hour, or overnight. To create a smoother sauce, blend the marinade liquids with the sun-dried tomatoes and re-toss with the vegetables, right before assembling the pies.

To make the "mashed potatoes", grind the nuts in a food processor, then add the cauliflower and the rest of the ingredients. Process until smooth. Scrape the sides of the processor with a spatula to ensure uniform blending.

Assemble the pies in individual tins, or layered in small bowls, with the "mashed potatoes" on top of the marinated vegetables. Allow the ingredients to reach room temperature, or heat in a warm oven for 1 hour, before serving. Garnish with paprika and parsley, or fresh hot peppers of your choice.

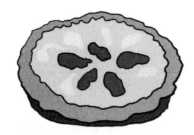

CHAPTER 5:
SUPER SIMPLE
SOUPS

Raw soups are super flavorful, and they can easily be warmed.

To warm a raw soup, use a double boiler so the temperature will rise slowly. Stirring often, warm the soup until it reaches no more than 119 degrees on a thermometer, or until it is warm to the touch.

I like making raw soups because they're fast, and generally easy to memorize. There are soups for every mood and occasion, from light cucumber soups to rich almond soups. Some, like Borscht and Chunky Tomato Chili, simply beg for creativity.

Once you try all the soups in this section, you'll be really good friends with your blender!

RAW FOODS FOR BUSY PEOPLE

⊘ MISO ALMOND SOUP

A quick enzyme boost, and easy to memorize.

1 Tb. unpasteurized miso of your choice

½ Tb. raw almond butter

1 cup warm or hot water

¼ cup chopped vegetables or mushrooms (optional)

1 chopped scallion, garnish

The vegetables will soften if you allow them to steep in hot water before stirring in the miso and nut butter.

⊘ Ⓑ RICH ALMOND SOUP

These are best warmed, and served with a light salad.

¼ cup raw almond butter

1 cup water

2 Tb. lemon or orange juice

1 Tb. Nama Shoyu

2 Tb. honey or agave syrup, or 3 pitted dates

2 scallions, minced

Cayenne, or chopped hot peppers, to taste

NUTTY BROCCOLI OR CAULIFLOWER SOUP:

Add 2 cups chopped broccoli or cauliflower

Omit sweetener, and add ½ tsp. curry powder or cumin

If you're using a whisk to make this soup, make sure the almond butter is at room temperature. If you're using dates, or the broccoli or cauliflower, you'll want to use a blender.

⊘ ⚙B CREAMY AVOCADO SOUP

Avocado = Smooth + Satisfying

2 large avocados

½ cup water

3 Tb. lemon juice

1 clove garlic, or ¼ tsp. garlic powder

Salt, or Bragg's liquid aminos, to taste

2 Tb. Italian seasoning

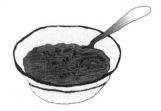

CITRUS SOUP: Add 1 cup orange juice + 1 tsp. jalapeno
MEXICAN SOUP: Omit Italian seasoning; add ½ tsp. each cumin and
black pepper, 1 tsp. minced jalapeno and 2 Tb. minced red onion
GREEN SOUP: Add 1 ½ cup chopped spinach OR broccoli

Combine all ingredients, and whisk or blend until smooth. If
using broccoli, you'll want to use a blender.

⚙B COOL CUCUMBER SOUP

This crisp, refreshing soup will soothe your digestion.

2 large cucumbers, peeled, seeded and chopped

¼ cup lemon juice

1 tsp. salt, or to taste

Water to thin

2 Tb. raw tahini, or 1 avocado (optional)

1 scallion, chopped

¼ cup fresh mint or dill

Combine all except the scallions and herbs, and whip until
smooth. Add the scallions and herbs and pulse blend, leaving
the greens in small pieces.

⊘ Ⓑ TANGY FRUIT SOUPS

Any fruit can be used for soup, with a bit of fresh mint.
Add nut butter or tahini for a richer base.

EZ FRUIT SOUP:

½ cup apple juice OR 1 whole apple, chopped

1-2 cups orange juice

¼ cup chopped fresh mint

Chopped hot peppers to taste (optional)

2 Tb. raw tahini, almond or cashew butter (optional)

REAL FRUIT SOUP:

Add 2 cups fruit of your choice to EZ Fruit Soup:

WALDORF SOUP:

Use 2 Tb. cashew butter or tahini with EZ Fruit Soup

Add 2 Tb. honey or 3 soft dates

Add 2 stalks of celery

Add ¼ cup each chopped parsley and scallions

FRUIT-FOR-DINNER SOUP:

Add 1 cup fresh carrot/celery/beet/pepper juice to EZ Fruit Soup

Add 1 fresh tomato, diced, and salt to taste

Blend or whisk the tahini or nut butters first, with the juice, before adding the rest of the ingredients. If using a whisk, it's best if your nut butters and juices are at room temperature. Float pieces of the fruit of your choice, or whole berries, in the soup. If using hot peppers, add conservatively and allow to marinate at least one hour in the refrigerator before adding more.
  Garnish with fresh mint.

⚙ FRESH TOMATO SOUPS

Use organic, ripe tomatoes. These recipes build on each other, so you can stay simple, or get crazy.

REAL TOMATO SOUP:

4 medium tomatoes

1 stalk celery

½ bell pepper, chopped

2 Tb. fresh basil, or 1 tsp. Italian seasoning

2 tsp. lemon juice

Salt, cayenne, and minced hot peppers to taste

CREAM OF TOMATO SOUP:

Add 1 avocado, and 2 tsp. maple or agave syrup

GO-GO GAZPACHO:

Blend a dash of cider vinegar with the Real Tomato Soup

Stir in minced zucchini, bell peppers and parsley

CHUNKY TOMATO CHILI:

Blend 1 cup BBQ Sauce (page 40) with the Real Tomato Soup

Blend in 2 tsp. chili powder, or hot peppers to taste

Mix in chunks of zucchini, bell peppers and green beans

Combine all ingredients of the Real Tomato Soup in a blender, and puree until desired consistency.

For the Cream of Tomato, Gazpacho, or Chili, blend the avocado and syrup, the vinegar, or the Barbecue Sauce and chili powder, respectively, with the Basic Tomato Soup recipe, and mix in the chopped vegetables by hand, where indicated.

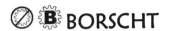 # BORSCHT

From traditional to modern, this is a sweet favorite the world over.

JUICE BAR BORSCHT:

2 cups fresh beet/carrot/celery/red pepper juice

2 Tb. raw tahini (at room temperature)

½ Tb. each lemon juice and Nama Shoyu

Chopped scallions

Finely chopped cabbage

Salt and pepper to taste

ANYTHING-YOU-WANT BORSCHT:

Juice Bar Borscht base

1 cup grated beets

1 red pepper or hot peppers, chopped

½ tsp. paprika

Chopped scallions

Chopped red or green cabbage

Chopped carrots

Sliced celery

Chopped apple

Diced avocado

Dollop of Sour Cream (page 39)

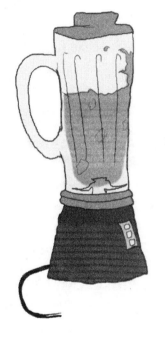

For Juice Bar Borscht, simply purchase fresh vegetable juice and whisk all ingredients together except scallions and cabbage. Float scallions and cabbage in the soup.

For Anything-You-Want Borscht, simply add grated beets, peppers and paprika to the Juice Bar Borscht base, and blend until smooth. Float any of the other ingredients (or any others you can think of!) in the soup.

⚙B FRESH CORN CHOWDER

I never knew corn didn't need to be cooked!

2 cups fresh corn, cut from the cob

1 cup water

¼ cup raw almond or cashew butter or tahini

2 scallions, minced

½ tsp. cumin OR pumpkin pie spice

Salt and pepper to taste

Minced red pepper to garnish

Chopped cilantro or sprouts to garnish

Blend the corn, water, nut butter or tahini, scallions and spice until smooth. Add salt and pepper to taste, and garnish with minced red pepper, and chopped cilantro or sprouts. This soup is great warmed (see page 43).

⚙B CURRIED COCONUT SOUP

This soup is well worth tackling a young coconut.

Meat and water from one young coconut

3 cups shredded carrots OR butternut squash

1 medium chopped onion

1 Tb. fresh lemon, lime or orange juice

1-2 Tb. curry powder

1 tsp. ground ginger

Pinch of cayenne, or minced hot peppers

Chopped cilantro to garnish

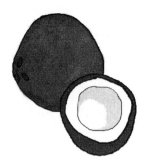

Blend all ingredients except the cilantro.
  Add cilantro just before serving.

CHAPTER 6:
DIP THIS,
DIP THAT

Dips are fun, there's no doubt about it. They are commonly a party food, are they not? From guacamole to salsas, nut spreads, garlicky pates, and fruit dips, these versatile dishes will give you that party feeling any day of the week. Furthermore, they're nutritious. Avocadoes, nuts and sprouted seeds are a great way to get high-quality protein and essential oils in your diet.

I have also included Nori Rolls in this chapter, which you can fill with the EZ Nori Filling (page 58), or with a Versatile Sunflower Pate (page 59).

So, go ahead! Dip vegetables, dip fruit, dip flax crackers and carrot chips. Throw yourself a party!

RAW FOODS FOR BUSY PEOPLE

⊘ AVOCADO STRAIGHT UP

Take advantage of the natural creaminess of avocado.

1 ripe avocado

½ lemon or lime

Salt and pepper or cayenne

Carrot sticks or Flax Crackers

Cut an avocado in half, and remove the pit. Squeeze fresh
lemon or lime juice over each half, and season with a dash of
salt and pepper or cayenne. Use carrot sticks or Flax Crackers
(page 68) to scoop the avocado right out of the skin.

⊘ Ⓓ QUICK AVOCADO PIZZA

Rich and nutritious, even when you're in a rush.

1 ripe avocado

Italian Seasoning

Italian or garlic-flavored Flax Crackers (page 68)

Chopped olives, onion, peppers, zucchini, and mushrooms

Spread fresh avocado on Flax Crackers you've bought or
dehydrated yourself, sprinkle with Italian Seasoning, and top
with veggies of your choice. *Voila!*

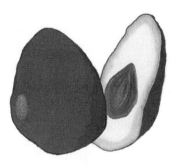

KITCHEN SINK GUACAMOLE

Perfect whether you only have a few minutes to whip something up, or you really want to show off.

2 ripe avocadoes

2-3 Tb. lemon or lime juice

1-2 cloves garlic, minced, or ¼ tsp. garlic powder

¼ c. minced red onion

Sea salt or Bragg's liquid aminos to taste

1 chopped tomato

OPTIONAL ADDITIONS:

Minced bell peppers, hot peppers, or cayenne

Chopped cilantro or parsley

Pine nuts or sunflower seeds

Sun-dried tomatoes, soaked 15 minutes and chopped

Chopped black olives

Basil, oregano and rosemary for an Italian flavor

GINGER PUMPKIN SEED GUACAMOLE:

Use ¼ cup orange juice instead of lemon or lime juice

Add 1 cup pumpkin seeds, soaked 10 minutes

Add ½ Tb. fresh grated ginger, or 1 tsp. ground ginger

Mash the avocado, then mix in citrus juice and spices. Fold in remaining ingredients, adding tomatoes last.

Serve Guacamole with dippin' veggies and Flax Crackers (page 68), or atop Carrot Chip Nachos (page 56). Serve it burrito-style in a cabbage or romaine lettuce leaf, with some salsa added. It's also a great accompaniment for Rawsome Rellenos (page 70).

Guacamole doesn't keep well, so if you make it ahead of time, squeeze citrus juice over the top, and leave the avocado pits in until right before serving time.

⊘ FRESH TOMATO SALSA

Use the best-quality, ripest tomatoes you can find.

1 ½ cups finely chopped tomatoes

1-2 Tb. lemon or lime juice

Minced peppers of your choice, to taste

2 cloves garlic, minced

1 tsp. sea salt, or to taste

½ cup chopped cilantro (optional)

SALSA VERDE:

Use green tomatoes, and include chopped parsley and basil

Toss all ingredients. If using hot peppers, add conservatively and let the salsa marinate for an hour before adding more.

Serve with sliced zucchini or Flax Crackers (page 68), or include in a pile of Carrot Chip Nachos (next page).

⊘ MANGO SALSA

Is it dinner or dessert?

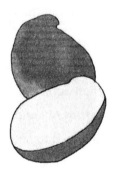

2 mangoes, chopped

1 small red onion, chopped

½ cup chopped cilantro

¼ cup lime or lemon juice

Minced peppers of your choice, to taste

1 tsp. sea salt, or to taste

Toss all ingredients. If using hot peppers, add conservatively and let the salsa marinate for an hour before adding more.

Serve with cucumber slices or Flax Crackers (page 68), or include in a pile of Carrot Chip Nachos (next page).

B CREAMY TOMATILLO SALSA

If you enjoy this as much as I do, you'll make it a staple.

4 tomatillos, chopped

1 minced jalapeno, or peppers of your choice

½-1 Tb. lime juice

¼ cup orange juice

½ tsp. salt, or to taste

1 ripe avocado

Blend all ingredients until desired consistency. If using hot peppers, add conservatively and let the salsa marinate for an hour before adding more.

Serve with Flax Crackers (page 68), or include in a pile of Carrot Chip Nachos (see below), or alongside Rawsome Rellenos (page 70).

F B CARROT CHIP NACHOS

Assemble the layers to your taste, and it's a fiesta!

Thick carrot ends, cut into round "chips"

Kitchen Sink Guacamole (page 54)

Fresh Tomato (previous page) or Creamy Tomatillo Salsa (see above)

Refried Almonds (page 60), or Mexican Pate (page 59)

Chopped tomatoes, lettuce and cilantro

Minced jalapeno, or hot peppers of your choice

Sweet carrots go very well with guacamole, dips, and salsas, so make this dish as simple or decadent as you wish. For a family or a party, make everything, including Flax Crackers (page 68), and call it a smorgasbord!

⊘ ⚙ INSTANT CINNAMON FRUIT DIP

Simply heavenly.

½ cup cashew or macadamia butter, or tahini

½ cup orange juice or water

¼ cup honey or agave syrup OR ½ cup soft dates

1 tsp. vanilla extract

1 Tb. cinnamon or pumpkin pie spice

½ tsp. orange zest

Blend or whisk nut butter with orange juice or water until smooth and creamy. Add the honey or agave syrup, or the dates two at a time, and then add the rest of the ingredients. Add more juice or water, until the dip reaches desired consistency.

If using a whisk, make sure your nut butter is at room temperature, and use honey or agave syrup.

Serve with sliced fruit. This dip is particularly good with tropical fruits, like banana and mango.

⚙ VERY BERRY FRUIT DIP

You won't believe what's in it.

1 ripe banana

½ ripe avocado (yup, avocado)

1 ½ cups mixed berries, fresh or frozen

1-2 Tb. lemon or orange juice

1-2 tsp. lemon or orange zest

1 Tb. honey or maple syrup, or ½ Tb. date sugar

Chopped fresh mint, or a pinch of dried mint

Pinch of sea salt

Blend all ingredients until smooth and creamy.

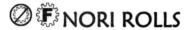 NORI ROLLS

Fresh and tasty, and easier than you think.

Raw nori sheets

EZ Nori Filling (see below), OR

Sweet & Sour Carrot Pate (next page)

Thin strips of carrot, cucumber and bell pepper

Slices of avocado

Sprouts of your choice

Shredded cabbage or lettuce (optional)

Chopped cilantro (optional)

Cut a large sheet of nori in half. Spread about 3 Tb. of your filling of choice along one of the narrow ends, ½ inch from the edge. Lay all your veggies on top of the filling, and roll the nori away from you, sealing the edge with a little water at the other end.
   Serve with Nama Shoyu and wasabi. *Itadakimasu!*

EZ NORI FILLING

Machine-free for quick preparation.

1/3 cup raw tahini or almond butter, at room temperature

3 Tb. unpasteurized miso of your choice

1 Tb. honey or agave syrup

1 clove garlic, minced, or 1/8 tsp. garlic powder

½ tsp. powdered ginger

¼ cup scallions, minced

1 Tb. Nama Shoyu, or more to taste

Mix all ingredients. Use in Nori Hand Rolls (see above), or for dippin' veggies.

F B VERSATILE SUNFLOWER PATE

A smooth, protein-packed basic pate.

2 cups sunflower seeds, sprouted (see page 32)

2 Tb. raw tahini

½ cup lemon juice

1-2 Tb. Nama Shoyu

1 large clove garlic, minced, or ¼ tsp. garlic powder

¼ cup chopped scallions

Pinch of cayenne

You can sprout your own sunflower seeds, or buy them from a health food store. If you're short on time, you can simply soak the seeds for 30 minutes before using.

Put all ingredients into a food processor with an S-blade and process until smooth, occasionally scraping the sides of the food processor with a spatula to ensure uniform blending. A blender can be used instead if you add water to thin the pate.

Use as a dip for veggies or Flax Crackers (page 68); to stuff celery sticks, avocadoes, tomatoes, or bell peppers; or as a base for one of the variations below.

Asian Pate: Mix in by hand 1 cup (total) of chopped veggies of your choice, including red onions, bell pepper, celery, bok choy, parsley, and/or cilantro. Mix in a little Citrus Ginger Marinade to bind the ingredients.

Mexican Pate: Substitute limejuice for lemon juice. Mix in by hand ½ cup each minced carrots, celery, zucchini, red onion, and chopped cilantro. Add 2 tsp. marjoram or thyme, and cayenne or minced hot peppers to taste. Use as a dip, or to stuff Rawsome Rellenos (page 70).

Sweet & Sour Carrot Pate: Mix in by hand 2-3 Tb. minced red onion, and 1 cup of carrot pulp, which you can procure from your nearest fresh juice bar. Add 1-2 Tb. fresh grated ginger and additional lemon juice and cayenne to taste. Use as a dip, or as a filling for Nori Rolls (previous page).

⚙️ REFRIED ALMONDS

So rich and nutty, it almost tastes cooked.

1 cup almonds, soaked 8-12 hours

½ cup lemon juice

1-2 cloves garlic, minced, or ¼ tsp. garlic powder

¼ cup sun-dried tomatoes, soaked 15 minutes, chopped

¼ cup red onion

1 tsp. each cumin, coriander and paprika

Pinch of cayenne

Sea salt to taste

Put all ingredients into a food processor with an S-blade. Process until smooth, or until the consistency of a traditional bean dip. Add a little water if needed.

Serve with dippin' veggies or Flax Crackers (page 68), or include in a pile of Carrot Chip Nachos (page 56).

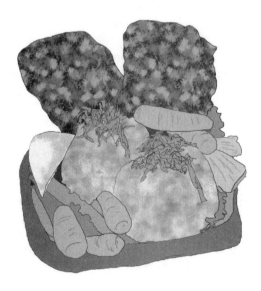

CHAPTER 7:
DEHYDRATION
FOR THE ROAD

Machine-free dehydration is possible, but only if you live in a *very* hot climate and can dry your food in the sun! As for the rest of us...

If I were to recommend any machine for busy people, it would be a dehydrator.

Dried foods are extremely convenient for people on the go, since they'll keep well in a desk drawer, glove compartment or backpack.

Using a dehydrator is easy and foolproof. Simply set the temperature to 105 degrees, put the food in, and turn the machine on. The recommended drying times are extremely flexible; I've forgotten about my dehydrating food for up to an extra twelve hours, and all was well.

By dehydrating your own foods, you'll be able to avoid commercially dried foods, which are cooked at high temperatures and often include added oil, sweeteners, chemicals and preservatives.

You can buy a simple dehydrator for only around $40-80 from Nesco. See page 88 for mail-order resources, or check your local appliance sources. Order some extra solid drying sheets too, which will be necessary for drying fruit leather, flax crackers and cookies.

RAW FOODS FOR BUSY PEOPLE

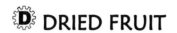 DRIED FRUIT

It doesn't get any simpler than this.

Fruit of your choice, sliced

Use literally any fruit you'd like. Bananas and apples are easy. Strawberries, mango and kiwis are especially tasty.

Fill your dehydrator trays with sliced fruit of your choice. Turn your dehydrator on, and allow fruit to dry for 8-12 hours or more.

Use solid dehydrator sheets when drying small fruit, like blueberries. Otherwise, use the slotted trays.

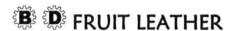 FRUIT LEATHER

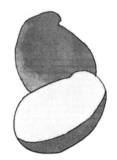

Let your imagination run wild!

2 cups of fruit

1 cup of juice or water

Put fruit of your choice into a blender with 1 cup of liquid, such as water, apple juice, grape juice, orange juice, or coconut water. Add a dash of sea salt. Liquefy until smooth, pour out onto solid dehydrator sheets, and dehydrate until dry, about 12-20 hours.

Sample Variations:
Apple or Pear Cinnamon Leather: 2 peeled and cored apples or pears, with 1 cup of apple juice or water, and 1 tsp. of cinnamon.
Mixed Berry Leather: Blend 2 cups of fresh or frozen berries with 1 cup of apple juice, grape juice, or water.
Tropical Fruit Leather: Blend 2 cups of mango, pineapple, banana, and/or kiwis with 1 cup of orange juice or water. Fresh young coconut meat, and young coconut water can be added as well.

⚙ SWEET SEED BARS

Sticky sweet and perfectly portable.

2 cups sesame/hemp/sunflower/pumpkin seed mix

5-6 Tb. Raw honey, or agave or maple syrup

Pinch of sea salt

VARIATION 1: Add 1-2 Tb. Lemon or orange juice

VARIATION 2: Add ½ Tb. Vanilla extract and ½ tsp. cinnamon

Soak seeds for 10 minutes before using. Mix all ingredients together with your hands. Shape into thin bars on solid dehydrator sheets. Dehydrate 8-12 hours, or until dry enough to remove from the solid sheets. Move bars to slotted dehydrator trays, and dehydrate for another 4-8 hours, or until dry on all sides.

When mixing the batch, wet your hands to prevent too much sticking. A wet, stiff rubber spatula may be used to shape the bars on the dehydrator sheets.

⚙ CITRUS ZESTS

Keep these around and sprinkle them on everything.

Fresh grated rind of lemon, lime or orange

Any time you're going to be juicing a few lemons, limes or oranges, consider making zest from the rind.

Finely grate the outer rind of your citrus fruit, before juicing it, and place the shavings on a solid dehydrator sheet. Dehydrate for about an hour, or until dry. For a fine consistency, you can grind the dried zest in a seed or coffee grinder. Either way, it's great to have around when you need it, and it makes an attractive garnish too.

⚙ NUT BUTTER COOKIES

To make this recipe without a food processor, buy your nuts already ground, or just use dried coconut. Otherwise, you can use a food processor to grind the nuts.

3 cups ground nuts and/or dried coconut

½ cup raw almond or cashew butter, at room temperature

¾ cup maple syrup or honey

2 Tb. olive or flaxseed oil

1 Tb. vanilla extract

Pinch of sea salt

CAROB COOKIES: Add ¼ cup carob powder

SPICE COOKIES: Add 1 Tb. cinnamon and ½ Tb. nutmeg

BANANA COOKIES: Replace 1 cup nuts with dried banana

Mix all ingredients by hand or with a food processor. Shape into cookies (see below), and place on solid dehydrator sheets. Dehydrate for 8-12 hours, and then move cookies to slotted dehydrator trays. Dehydrate for another 4-8 hours or more, until dry on the outside.

If you're as lazy (er... I mean busy) as I am, you'll like this trick I use for shaping cookies. If your cookie dough turns out too stiff or dry, shaping the cookies will require either rolling and re-rolling the dough out between wax paper sheets and cutting it, or shaping it into unattractive wads with your hands. My shortcut includes adding water to the cookie dough until it's soft enough to be formed into pliable balls. I then place a solid dehydrator sheet in front of me on the counter and throw each ball of dough at the sheet. They splat into perfect cookie shapes, with no trouble at all! Adding the extra water makes for extra drying time, of course, but I don't mind waiting. *That's* effortless.

CRISPY ONION TOPPERS

These are great on salads, or to top off any vegetable dish. Use on top of the Barbecue Portobello on page 35.

Two large onions

1 cup Nama Shoyu

1/3 cup olive oil

Garlic powder, cayenne or Chinese 5-spice (optional)

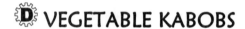

Slice onion into ringlets and marinate in tamari, olive oil and spices, for 1 to 8 hours. Remove ringlets from marinade and place on solid dehydrator sheets for 12-20 hours, or until crisp.

VEGETABLE KABOBS

Serve with a salad, the Barbecue Portobello, or Nori Rolls.

Zucchini or yellow squash

Mushrooms of any kind

Peppers and Onions

Cherry tomatoes

Cauliflower and Broccoli

Carrots

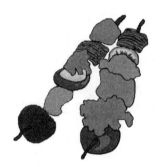

Cut vegetables into large chunks. Use any marinade of your choice from Chapter 4.

Marinate the vegetables for at least 2 hours at room temperature, or overnight in the refrigerator. Skewer your veggies, and dehydrate for up to 24 hours, or until as soft as desired. To reheat, return cold Kabobs to the dehydrator for 1 hour.

⚙ FLAVORED NUTS & SEEDS

A great alternative to popcorn, and easier to sneak into the cinema.

2-4 cups nuts and seeds of your choice

SALTY NUT MARINADE:

Nama Shoyu, or sea salt dissolved in water

Crushed garlic, or garlic powder (optional)

Crushed red pepper or cayenne (optional)

HONEY NUT MARINADE:

(for 2 cups of nuts and seeds)

¼ cup honey, agave or maple syrup

1 ½ Tb. vanilla extract

Pinch of salt

Cinnamon and nutmeg (optional)

Chili powder (optional)

Cover nuts and seeds with the Salty Marinade, or toss with the Sweet Marinade. Allow to marinate for 30 minutes to 24 hours (the longer the stronger). Spread on mesh or solid dehydrator sheets, depending on the size of the seed or nut, and dehydrate for 12-24 hours, or until dry.

If using the Sweet Marinade, soak the nuts or seeds for at least 10-30 minutes before tossing. Ideally, nuts and seeds should be thoroughly soaked, so if you have the time, soak almonds and sunflower seeds for 8-12 hours; walnuts and pumpkin seeds for 2-4 hours; cashews for 30 minutes; and all other nuts 4-6 hours.

Serve as a snack, or toss with a green salad, coleslaw, or Pineapple Waldorf Salad (page 30).

⚙ FLAX CRACKERS

Try this experiment: Soak ¼ cup of flax seeds in ½ cup of water for 3 hours. Stick your finger in it. Now you know why flax crackers are so easy to make: It's the goo!

2 cups flax seeds

4 cups water

Salt, spices or vegetables (see below)

½ cup sesame or hemp seeds (optional)

For a blender-free version, soak flax seeds as described above, spread the flax seed goo onto solid dehydrator sheets, and sprinkle with your choice of salt, garlic powder, Italian seasonings, cayenne, or Chinese 5-spice.

For more complex flavors, you can use a blender to liquefy the veggies and spices of your choice in the water, before adding to the flax seeds for soaking (see below). If using wet vegetables, like tomatoes, reduce the water to 3 cups.

Dehydrate for 8-12 hours, and then move crackers to slotted trays and dehydrate for 4-8 hours more, or until crisp.

A stiff spatula works well to spread the flax goo onto the dehydrator sheets. If you don't have enough solid dehydrator sheets for all the goo you've got, you can spread the goo onto pieces of waxed paper. If you use waxed paper, however, you must watch your drying time carefully and remove the crackers from the paper after about 3-4 hours. If the crackers are left on waxed paper for too long, they'll be stubbornly stuck together.

Sample Variations:
Mexican Flax Crackers: Blend water with fresh tomatoes, cilantro, lime juice, peppers, garlic, and salt.
Italian Flax Crackers: Blend water with tomatoes, zucchini, garlic, Italian seasoning, fresh basil, olives, bell peppers, and salt.
Asian Flax Crackers: Blend water with Nama Shoyu, lemon juice, cilantro, peppers, garlic, and Chinese 5-spice.

🄵 🄳 PESTO-STUFFED VEGETABLES

These make great hors d'oeuvres.
Oh, and a good pesto deserves fresh garlic.

1/3 cup pine nuts, soaked 10-20 minutes

2-3 cloves fresh garlic, minced

½ cup chopped parsley

½ cup chopped fresh basil

1 Tb. olive oil

Pinch of salt

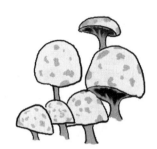

SPINACH PESTO: Substitute ½ cup of chopped spinach for ¼ cup of the parsley

Mushroom caps

Bell pepper chunks

Zucchini or yellow squash rounds

Grind the pine nuts in a food processor, or pound them in a mortar. Add the garlic and olive oil to the nuts, and process or pound until blended. Gradually add the greens and pulse chop or pound until finely chopped. Salt to taste. Put a dollop of pesto onto each vegetable piece, and dehydrate for 3-4 hours.

Regularly scrape the sides of the food processor with a spatula to ensure uniform blending and consistency. You can make the pesto ahead and allow it to marinate overnight.

If another item is dehydrating at the same time, put the pesto veggies on the bottom. Pesto drippings don't taste very well on cookies!

If serving as hors d'oeuvres, drizzle each piece with olive oil, garnish with whole pine nuts, and serve with whole raw olives.

⚙F ⚙D RAWSOME RELLENOS

Muy bien!

One batch of Mexican Pate (page 59)

Anaheim peppers, or peppers of your choice

Zucchini "boats"

Slice your peppers down the middle lengthwise, or bell peppers into three or four strips, along the indentations lengthwise. Remove the seeds. For zucchini, cut into wide strips and remove enough of the center to create indentations. Fill each pepper or zucchini strip with Mexican Pate, and dehydrate for 6-8 hours. To reheat, dehydrate cold Rellenos for one hour or more.

If you're not sure what kind of pepper to use, choose Anaheim peppers. You can use hotter ones if you're so inclined, or just use bell peppers or zucchini if you're a spice wimp. If you're serving guests, use a variety of peppers of various colors.

These are great served with cold Creamy Tomatillo Salsa, made on the mild side (page 55), or with Sour Cream (page 39).

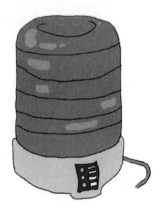

CHAPTER 8:
ALMOST EFFORTLESS DESSERTS

You could eat any of the following desserts for breakfast, lunch and dinner, and still be eating better than you ever have in your life.

Desserts are our friends. Our sweet tooth is natural: it is our innate propensity toward fresh fruit. After all, if you're in a natural setting, and you have a sweet tooth, what do you reach for? Fruit, of course!

Unfortunately, our natural taste for sweet fruit is working against us in the modern world, since our taste buds have been exposed to artificial and concentrated sugars not found in nature.

But never fear. This chapter will have you on a healthy course in no time. How about some vitamins, enzymes, fiber and living water with your (natural) sugar? What a concept!

⊘ CINNAMON STEWED FRUIT

Forget the cooked, lifeless version.
This marinated fruit is full of natural flavor.

4 ripe apples, pears, or peaches, sliced

2 Tb. lemon juice

1 tsp. lemon zest

½ cup apple juice

1 Tb. cinnamon or pumpkin pie spice

1 Tb. agave or maple syrup (optional)

½ cup raisins or currants (optional)

¼ cup chopped or ground pecans or nuts (optional)

Toss all ingredients and allow to marinate for at least an hour, allowing the lemon juice to soften the fruit.
   Top with Whipped Cashew Cream (page 82) for an additional dimension of flavor.

⊘ BERRIES ROMANOFF

Traditionally made with a dash of Cointreau liqueur.

1 pint fresh strawberries or mixed berries

½ cup orange juice

½ tsp. orange zest

2 Tb. date sugar or agave syrup

½ tsp. cinnamon (optional)

Chopped almonds to garnish

Simply marinate the strawberries for an hour or more, and enjoy.
   Top this dessert off with Orange Cashew Cream (page 82) for a truly decadent treat.

PINEAPPLE CARROTS

Consider this a machine-free carrot cake!

2-3 cups grated carrots

½ cup each chopped pineapple and raisins

1 Tb. lemon juice

½ cup pineapple or orange juice

1 tsp. each cinnamon, nutmeg and powdered ginger

Dash of vanilla extract

4-6 fresh pineapple rings

¼ cup each chopped walnuts and parsley, to garnish

Toss all ingredients except the pineapple rings and garnishes, and marinate for at least an hour, allowing the juices to soften the carrots.

Serve the marinated carrots on top of each pineapple ring, and garnish. Add Lemon Whipped Cream (page 82) if desired.

SWEET SPREADS

Lick it off your hands, and feel like a kid again.

Raw almond or cashew butter, OR

¼ cup tahini mashed with 1 Tb. honey or agave syrup

Celery or carrot sticks

Apple slices, with fresh berries

Banana, with Carob Sauce (page 76)

A batch of Nut Butter Cookies (page 65)

Smear nut butter and sweetened tahini on absolutely anything.

⊘ NIRVANA BARS

Roll up your sleeves for this one!

4 cups ground walnuts

1 cup ground cashews, macadamias or almonds

1 cup sunflower and/or pumpkin seeds

1 cup dried coconut (optional)

½ cup raw carob powder (optional)

1 cup almond butter (at room temperature)

½ cup maple syrup, or more to taste

¼ cup flaxseed oil

Pinch of sea salt

Toss the nuts, seeds, coconut and carob powder together first. Whip the almond butter, maple syrup, oil and salt together separately, either with a whisk or in a food processor. Using your hands, mash all the ingredients together until the nut mixture is completely coated.

The mixture should be fairly dry while you're working with it, so spend some time really mashing it all together. If the mixture is too wet, it won't stand up in solid bars after refrigerating.

Refrigerate in a short, rectangular container for at least 3 hours, and then cut into bars. It's raw candy!

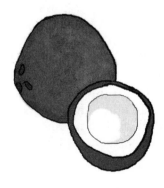

⚙️ INSTANT CREAMER

Enjoy in your favorite tea, or over fruit or raw granola.

1 Tb. raw cashew butter OR ¼ cup cashews, soaked 30 min.

½ - ¾ cup water

INSTANT ALMOND MILK:

1 Tb. raw almond butter

½ cup water

Blend until smooth and creamy.

    This makes a healthy creamer for any beverage. You can also pour it over fresh strawberries, bananas or peaches, or purchase raw granola from one of the companies listed on pages 87-88.

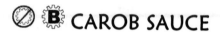 CAROB SAUCE

This goes well on just about anything.

1 cup raw carob powder

½ cup pitted soft dates, soaked 10 minutes

½ cup maple or agave syrup

2 Tb. olive or coconut oil (optional)

2 Tb. vanilla extract (optional)

MEXICAN CAROB SAUCE: Add 2 tsp. cinnamon

A blender works best with this sauce, though you can use a whisk if you substitute additional syrup for the dates, and use the olive or coconut oil and some elbow grease. Add a little water if the sauce is too thick.

⊘ ⚙ Ⓑ CREAMY PUDDINGS

Avocado, banana and soft nuts make creamy puddings.

AVOCADO BASED PUDDING:

1 ripe avocado

1 ripe banana OR ¼ cup pitted dates, soaked 10 minutes

½ cup berries OR ¼ cup raw carob powder

2 tsp. vanilla extract

BANANA BASED PUDDING:

1 ripe banana

6 dates, soaked up to 30 minutes

2-3 peaches, or meat and water from one young coconut

2 tsp. vanilla extract

1 tsp. cinnamon (optional)

NUT BASED PUDDING:

1 cup cashews soaked 30 min., or almonds soaked 8 hrs.

½ cup water, orange juice or coconut water

1 ripe banana OR ¼ cup pitted dates, soaked 10 minutes

½ cup dried or fresh coconut (optional)

Sliced banana or fresh berries of your choice

For the avocado and banana based puddings, simply whip up all ingredients in a blender, or mash and whisk by hand if not using dates. Use a spatula to scrape the sides of the blender a few times during blending.

For the nut-based puddings, blend the nuts and water or juice first, until truly smooth, before adding the rest of the ingredients.

Top with Whipped Cashew Cream (page 82) if desired.

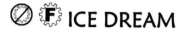 ICE DREAM

A natural, frozen treat.

2 cups frozen fruit of your choice

2 Tb. sweetener of your choice

¼ cup raw carob powder (optional)

¼ cup fruit juice OR Instant Creamer or Almond Milk (optional) (page 76)

Softer fruits work best, such as bananas, strawberries, peaches and mangoes.

Peel your fruit, if desired, before cutting it into small pieces and freezing.

Add sweetener, carob powder and/or nut milk to the frozen fruit and mash either with a potato masher or in a food processor. Enjoy right away or re-freeze.

To make a sundae, top with Carob Sauce (page 76), Whipped Cashew Cream (page 82) and chopped nuts.

B HALVAH SHAKE

Sesame tahini makes for a rich and creamy shake.

2-3 Tb. tahini

1 Tb. almond butter

1 fresh or frozen ripe banana

2 dates, or 1 Tb. honey or agave syrup

Dash of vanilla extract

3-4 Tb. raw carob powder (optional)

½-1 cup water

Blend all ingredients until smooth and creamy. Add a few ice cubes if desired. *Tip:* Peel bananas before freezing.

⚙️B CARAMEL APPLE SHAKE

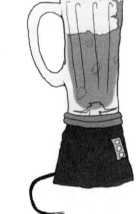

Decadence in a glass.

1 apple, cut in chunks

1 cup apple juice

2-3 Tb. almond butter

2 Tb. maple syrup, OR 3 pitted soft dates

Dash of cinnamon and nutmeg

1 ripe banana (optional)

ORANGE PECAN SHAKE:

Use ½ cup pecans instead of almond butter

Add ¼ cup raisins soaked in ¼ cup orange juice

Add a dash of orange zest

Blend all ingredients until smooth.

⚙️B JORDAN'S POWER SHAKE

When you want something heavier, or for after a workout.

Meat and water from one young coconut

1-2 Tb. protein or supplement powder of your choice

¼ - ½ cup orange juice

2 Tb. almond butter (optional)

Dash of vanilla extract (optional)

Blend all ingredients until smooth.

⚙ DATE NUT LOGS

Now, you'll know how to make your own.

1 cup pitted dates, soaked up to 30 minutes

½ cup dates, dried apricots or figs, soaked 30 minutes

1 cup pecans, walnuts or almonds, ground

1 cup dried coconut

1 tsp. cinnamon or pumpkin pie spice

Grind dry nuts in a food processor, or buy your nuts ground. Add coconut first, and then cinnamon and vanilla. Finally, add dates and other dried fruit a few pieces at a time. Shape batter into small logs ½-3/4 inch thick, and roll in dried coconut. Chill until stiff.

⚙ PARTY BALLS

Eat these ungarnished, or dress them up for a party.

1 cup almonds, ground

2 Tb. pine nuts or cashews or macadamias, ground

½ cup dried shredded coconut

¼ cup raw almond butter

¼ cup honey or syrup, or more to hold balls together

CAROB BALLS: Add 1 cup carob powder + ¼ cup water

Combine the nuts, coconut, and carob powder, if using, in a food processor with an S-blade. Mix the almond butter, sweetener, and water if needed, separately, and then add to the dry ingredients. The dough should be fairly dry, but wet enough to hold together when rolled into balls. If you're dressing them up, roll each ball in carob powder, or finely ground coconut or almonds. Refrigerate several hours, until firm.

B VANILLA-CACAO LATTE

Use raw cacao for a new-fashioned cappuccino! Use a nut-milk bag for extra smoothness.

½ cup raw cacao beans, soaked overnight in 2 cups water

2 Tb. cashew, macadamia or almond butter

2 Tb. tahini or hemp seed butter

2-3 Tb. agave syrup or honey

1 tsp. pure vanilla extract

Pinch of sea salt

2 Tb. powdered maca (optional)

FLAVORED LATTE: Replace 1 cup water with strong tea, such as mint, orange or raspberry

RICH CHOCOLATE MILK: Use ½ cup raw carob powder, or more to taste, in place of cacao beans

If, like many busy people, you have a taste for specialty coffee drinks, you'll enjoy this rich, healthy alternative.

Combine soaked cacao beans and water with the nut and seed butters, and blend for several minutes. Put this mixture through a nut-milk bag or a fine strainer to remove the solid pieces. Take your time with the nut-milk bag, if using, squeezing gently so as not to tear it. Return the liquid to the blender, adding the rest of the ingredients, including sweetener, vanilla, salt, and maca, if using. Blend well. The heat of a Vita-Mix will warm the beverage, or you can warm it using a double boiler.

Interestingly, raw cacao does not cause the excitement of the nervous and circulatory systems, or the accelerated pulse, often caused by roasted cacao. Enjoy your cacao latte in good health!

To make Rich Chocolate Milk, no soaking is required. Simply blend all ingredients. Using a nut-milk bag is still recommended for a super-smooth beverage.

🅑 WHIPPED CASHEW CREAM

One taste of this and you'll never go back to dairy.

1 ½ cups cashews, soaked 30 minutes

½ cup water, or juice to flavor (see below)

4-5 dates, soaked 30 minutes

1 tsp. vanilla or almond extract

ORANGE CREAM: Use orange juice + a dash of orange zest

APPLE CREAM: Use apple juice + a dash of cinnamon

LEMON CREAM: Use 1/3 cup lemon juice + ¼ cup honey or syrup

COCONUT CREAM: Use coconut water + extra vanilla

In a blender, combine the nuts and water or juice first. Blend until smooth and creamy. Add the dates two at a time, and then the remaining ingredients. Use a spatula to scrape the sides of the blender a few times during blending. Be patient, and make sure it gets real smooth.

This is a healthy topping for any dessert, or to complement fresh berries or sliced bananas.

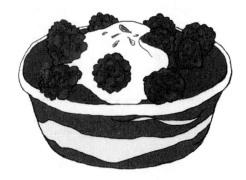

RESOURCES

•

INDEX

RAW FOODS FOR BUSY PEOPLE

SUGGESTED READING

RAW INSPIRATION

Boutenko, Victoria. *12 Steps to Raw Foods: How to End Your Addiction to Cooked Food.*
Cobb, Brenda. *The Living Foods Lifestyle.*
Cousens, Gabriel, M.D. *Conscious Eating.*
Halfmoon, Hygeia, Ph.D. *Primal Mothering in a Modern World.*
Malkmus, George. *God's Way to Ultimate Health.*
Miller, Susie & Knowler, Karen. *Feel-good Food.*
Monarch, Matthew. *Raw Spirit.*
Nison, Paul. *Raw Knowledge II: Interviews with Health Achievers.*
Owen, Bob. *Roger's Recovery from AIDS.*
Szekely, Edmond Bordeaux, trans. *The Essene Gospel of Peace.*
Wolfe, David. *Eating for Beauty.*

RAW FOOD NUTRITION

American Natural Hygiene Society. *The Natural Hygiene Handbook.*
Boutenko, Victoria. *Green for Life.*
Cousens, Gabriel, M.D. *Depression Free for Life.*
Diamond, Harvey. *You Can Prevent Breast Cancer!*
Diamond, Harvey and Marilyn. *Fit for Life II: Living Health.*
Francis, Raymond, R.N.C., M.Sc.. *Never Be Sick Again: Health is a Choice, Learn How to Choose It*
Howell, Edward, Dr. *Enzyme Nutrition.*
Meyerowitz, Steve. *Sprouts: The Miracle Food.*
Meyerowitz, Steve. *Wheatgrass: Nature's Finest Medicine.*
Shelton, Herbert M., Dr. *Natural Hygiene: The Pristine Way of Life.*
Walker, Norman, D.Sc., Ph.D. *Become Younger.*
Wigmore, Ann, Dr. *The Hippocrates Diet and Health Program.*

NATURAL FITNESS

Arlin, Stephen. *Raw Power!: Building Strength and Muscle Naturally.*
Brazier, Brendan. *Thrive: A guide to optimal health and performance through plant-based whole foods.*
La Lanne, Jack. *Revitalize Your Life.*

COLON HEALTH AND DETOXIFICATION

Anderson, Richard, N.D. *Cleanse and Purify Thyself.*
Burroughs, Stanley. *The Master Cleanser.*
Krok, Morris. *Golden Path to Rejuvenation.*
Meyerowitz, Steve. *Juice Fasting and Detoxification.*
Morse, Robert, N.D. *The Detox Miracle Sourcebook.*
Walker, Norman, D.Sc., Ph.D. *Colon Health: The Key to a Vibrant Life.*

RAW RECIPE BOOKS

Baird, Lori, ed. *The Complete Book of Raw Foods.*
Calabro, Rose Lee. *Living in the Raw.*
Cornbleet, Jennifer. *Raw Food Made Easy.*
Cousens, Gabriel, M.D., and the Tree of Life Café Chefs. *Rainbow Green Live Food Cuisine.*
Juliano. *Raw: The Uncook Book.*
Levin, James, M.D. *Vibrant Living.*
Malkmus, Rhonda J. *Recipes for Life from God's Garden.*
Markowitz, Elysa. *Warming Up to Living Foods.*
Mars, Brigitte. *Rawsome!*
Rhio. *Hooked on Raw.*
Romano, Rita. *Dining in the Raw.*
Shannon, Nomi. *The Raw Gourmet.*
Trotter, Charlie, and Klein, Roxanne. *Raw.*
Underkoffler, Renee Loux. *Living Cuisine: The Art and Spirit of Raw Foods.*

VIDEOS & DVD'S

Cohen, Alissa. *Living on Live Foods.*
Cousens, Gabriel, M.D. *Rainbow Green Live Food Cuisine.*
Day, Lorraine, M.D. *Cancer Doesn't Scare Me Anymore!*
Day, Lorraine, M.D. *You Can't Improve on God.*
Maerin, Jordan. *Raw Foods for Busy People: The Video.*
Malkmus, George. *How to Eliminate Sickness.*

RAW LIFESTYLE MAGAZINES

Health Science, (813) 855-6607 healthscience.org
Just Eat An Apple, justeatanapple.com
Living Nutrition, (707) 829-0362 livingnutrition.com

ONLINE RESOURCES

alissacohen.com: Instructional classes and videos, books.
anhs.org: American Natural Hygiene Society website.
audreyrochester.com: Snacks, cookies, chips, breads.
beyondhealth.com: Raymond Francis, healthy olive oil.
davidwolfe.com: Updated lists of raw restaurants.
essenespirit.com: Information about the Essene teachings.
goodmoodfood.com: Order snacks and crackers.
goraw.org: Granola, flax crackers, energy bars.
living-foods.com: Internet educational community.
rawbakery.com: Gourmet desserts.
rawfamily.com: Instructional videos, books, food items.
rawfood.com: Nature's First Law superstore.
raw-pleasure.com: International raw directory.
sunorganic.com: Dried fruit, nuts, olives, flax products.
thegardendiet.com: Retreats and professional resources.
therawworld.com: Dr. Fred Bisci's online resource.

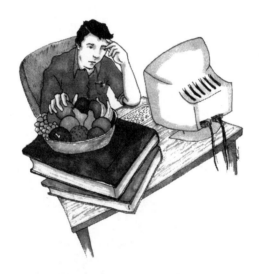

MAIL ORDER RESOURCES

Fingerhut: Appliances. 1-800-208-2500
Freeland Foods: Granola, snack bars. (619) 286-2446
Living Tree: Nut butters, etc. 1-800-260-5534
Mountain Home Basics: Appliances. 1-800-572-9549
Nature's First Law: All things raw. 1-888-RAW-FOOD
Sun Organic Farm: Nuts, flax, olives. 1-888-269-9888

RAW FOOD HEALING CENTERS

Creative Health Institute, Union City, Michigan
    creativehealthinstitute.us 1-866-426-1213
Hallelujah Acres (Christian), North Carolina and Ontario
    hacres.com 1-877-743-2589
Happy Oasis, Prescott, Arizona
    happyoasis.com (928) 708-0784
Hippocrates Institute, West Palm Beach, Florida
    hippocratesinst.org (561) 471-8876
Living Foods Institute, Atlanta, Georgia
    livingfoodsinstitute.com 1-800-844-9876
National Health Association, various locations
    www.anhs.org/community.htm (813) 855-6607
Optimum Health Institute, San Diego and Austin, Texas
    optimumhealth.org 1-800-993-4325
Sanoviv Medical Institute, Baja Coast of Mexico
    sanoviv.com 1-800-726-6848
Tanglewood Wellness Center, Frederick, Maryland
    tanglewoodwellnesscenter.com (301) 898-8901
Tree of Life Rejuvenation Center, Patagonia, Arizona
    www.treeoflife.nu (520) 394-2520

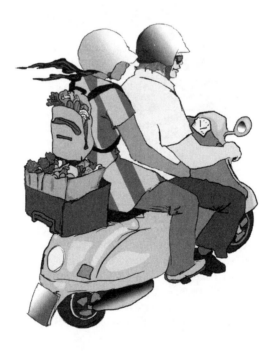

RECIPE INDEX

Jordan Maerin

Love. Health. Creativity. Contribution.

Visit the website for busy people:

www.rawfoodsforbusypeople.com

Includes:
Author Bio
Book Ordering Information
Original Articles
Updates on Future Projects
Sungazing Journal

Plus:
Quick Web Links
to the resources and products you need most!

ABOUT THE AUTHOR

Jordan Maerin holds a degree in Philosophy from Michigan State University. She is a raw food enthusiast, nature-lover and sungazer living in southern California.

OTHER TITLES

Raw Foods for Busy People: The Video
Alimentos Crudos para La Gente Ocupada

A RAW FOOD BLESSING

I give thanks for the raw nutrients in this food, which I digest and absorb easily.

I give thanks for the living energy of this food, and in accepting it, I align myself with the generous energies of the Earth and Sun.

I give thanks for the nourishment of this food, which I accept openly, joyfully and righteously.

I give thanks for the divine illusion of this food, representing as it does the infinite cosmic energy of which I am a part.

I give thanks for this food as a tool of my intention to manifest my own strong, vibrant, comfortable body.

NOTES

RAW FOODS FOR BUSY PEOPLE

NOTES

NOTES

RAW FOODS FOR BUSY PEOPLE